Skincare for Runners

TIPS AND TRICKS FOR THE EVERYDAY ATHLETE

Brooke A. Jackson, MD, FAAD
- Top Dermatologist
- Marathoner

joyla

be your best you

To my parents, who encouraged me to try
To my husband, whose ever-present support lets me fly
To my children, who are my why

© 2021 by Brooke A. Jackson, MD

All rights reserved. No part of this publication may be reproduced or transmitted in any form or by any means, electronic or mechanical, including photocopying, recording, or any other information storage and retrieval system, without the written permission of the publisher.

This publication also includes references to third-party trademarks, which are owned and may be registered by third parties whose products are mentioned in this publication.

Any and all unauthorized uses of these third-party marks are also prohibited.

Printed in the United States of America

Cover and interior designs by Jennifer Giandomenico

ISBN 978-1-952481-27-7

Library of Congress 2021911789

2   4   6   8   10   9   7   5   3   1   paperback

For information on bulk copies contact Jennifer@BrightCommunications.net

Bright
COMMUNICATIONS

BrightCommunications.net

Contents

Foreword

In 1996, when my husband Dave and I opened Fleet Feet in Chicago, we had no idea how many people we would meet and how interesting they would be. We did not expect to make friends and build lifelong bonds through the one common thread of running.

The day Dr. Brooke Jackson walked into our store, I had no idea that I would have a friend for life. Dr. Jackson brought a passion and a plan to the Chicago Running community. She helped us realize that we had a platform to educate runners and athletes on more than the products we sold. Passionate about skincare for those of us who were running outside in the sunshine and crazy Chicago weather every day, we soon began working together, setting up speaking engagements at club runs and running races with various training groups on Proper Skin Care for runners.

As I read this book, I could hear Dr. Jackson's voice in every word. The more technical information on the skin is written understandably. The chapter on sun protection removes much of the mystery of SPFs and the effects of the sun. The boxed sidebars and diagrams make the book a valuable reference tool. As I age and look to more holistic solutions in my life, I found the chapters on essential nutrition, healthy skin, and CBD incredibly useful for navigating these topics.

Skincare for Runners is a must-have for every outdoor athlete, whether you are a runner, walker, or simply spend time outside. This book is informative and a great reference tool for anyone who is embarking on a marathon journey. The pages are filled with skincare advice and practical, helpful tips for all aspects of the marathon journey. It is a reference tool that I will keep on my desk. You might ask, "Why not just Google it?" My answer is because I know Dr. Jackson, and I trust her answers, suggestions, and knowledge. She has run the miles, crossed the finish lines, and been a leader of athletes in Chicago's running community. You can see she is exceptionally well educated, and yes, she is a fantastic doctor, but as her friend, I can tell you firsthand about her passion for educating others and sharing her knowledge with the endurance athlete. She understands the athlete, and she also revels in the endurance sports lifestyle.

As you read the pages, think about the hours and hours that Dr. Jackson and I spent running together on the Chicago lakefront path and know that she genuinely and sincerely believes that her knowledge can make your journey more enjoyable, safer, and healthier.

—Lisa Zimmer
Owner, Fleet Feet Chicago

Introduction

I have been an athlete all my life. And while I will never bring home an Olympic medal and chances are good that no one will ever pay to see me participate in sports, my desire to stay active and participate in sports has never faltered.

I started swimming as a child and won a few medals in the backstroke, played field hockey and softball in high school, ran my first marathon in my thirties, and organized, directed, and coached a marathon-training group on the South Side of Chicago not long after that. Today, as a board-certified dermatologist and amateur athlete, I teach my patients and lecture to running groups about proper care for athlete's skin, sun safety, and skin cancer prevention.

I have many athletes in my practice, ranging from the middle-school athlete to the casual weekend golfer to the Olympic qualifier and professional athlete. I enjoy working with and helping athletes, especially runners, take care of their skin.

I wrote this book to provide information and guidance to the athlete in all of us.

Keep putting one foot in front of the other and you will get to the finish line. Run happy, run safe.

—Brooke A. Jackson, MD

Chapter 1
Your Skin

Skin is the largest and heaviest organ of your body. In an average-sized adult, the skin comprises about one-seventh of total body weight and, if stretched out, would span approximately 20 square feet. Just like each of your other organs, such as the heart, lungs, and kidneys, your skin plays a significant role in keeping you alive and maintaining your overall health.

Your skin serves as the barrier between you and the outside world. It prevents water loss and protects against harmful environmental elements such as bacteria, viruses, mold, parasites' and ultraviolet (UV) light damage. It also prevents your internal organs from seeping into the outside world. Simply put, your skin functions like a breathable, waterproof seal.

To understand the skin's function, you must first understand skin anatomy. Skin is composed of three layers of tissue: the epidermis, dermis, and subcutis.

The *epidermis* is the outermost layer. It provides a

Skin Cross-Section

sweat pore — ← hair shaft

melanocytes

sebaceous gland

epidermis

sweat gland

blood vessels

hair follicle

hair erector muscle

dermis

hypodermis

waterproof barrier seal from your environment, gives skin its color, and constantly generates new skin cells. New epidermal cells, called keratinocytes, are made in the lower portion of the epidermis and, over the course of 30 to 45 days, migrate from the bottom of the epidermis to the top of the epidermis, after which they fall off as dead skin. Millions of dead skin cells are shed each day.

The natural color of skin is determined by the amount of pigment produced. Skin pigment, or melanin, is produced by specialized epidermal cells called melanocytes, which are found in the lower portion of the epidermis. Everyone, regardless of skin color, has the same number of pigment-producing melanocytes. What differs and determines natural skin color is the level of activity and the size of pigment produced by melanocytes. Those with naturally darker skin have larger, more active melanocytes that produce pigment packages called melanosomes. These melanosomes are scattered throughout the epidermis, giving skin its darker hue. Those with fair skin have smaller, less active melanocytes and fewer melanosomes.

The *dermis* is the middle layer of the skin. It contains sweat and oil glands, hair follicles, and the blood supply of our skin. It also contains receptors for pain, pressure, and heat that are largely responsible for the sensations we experience. The upper portion of the dermis, called the *papillary dermis*, is made of connective tissue that creates unique identifying information about us, such as our fingerprints. The bottom portion of the dermis is known as the *reticular dermis*. It contains the protein fibers elastin and collagen, which provide strength and flexibility to our skin. Damage to this layer can result in scar formation. Excessive stretching of our skin during growth spurts, such as from weight gain, pregnancy, or adolescent growth, results in stretch marks.

The *subcutis* or *hypodermis* is the deepest layer of skin. It is a web of connective tissue, fat, and elastin functioning as glue to keep our skin attached to underlying muscle and bone. The fat of the subcutis helps us maintain our body temperature by providing insulation and cushioning for our muscles and bones.

Skin Functions

- Protective barrier
- Sensation
- Temperature regulation
- Storage and synthesis of nutrients

Chapter 2
Essential Nutrition for Healthy Skin

For skin to perform its many functions properly, it requires proper nutrition and hydration. A well-balanced diet will benefit your entire body, not just your skin. Chronic inflammation is the root of many disease processes. A plant-based diet will provide an excellent foundation for a well-balanced, anti-inflammatory diet. It is always better to eat whole foods in their natural state rather than processed or packaged foods.

Plant-Based Diet

Following a plant-based diet has many benefits. Naturally low in saturated fat and cholesterol-free, a plant-based

Rule of Thumb

Eat foods that come from the ground (fruit, vegetables, grains, legumes) and minimize those that come from a package.

Looking to learn more?
I recommend these two documentaries on Netflix:

- *Game Changers:* The benefits of plant-based diets for athletes are discussed in this documentary.
- *Forks Over Knives:* This documentary explains how food is medicine and how to adopt a plant-based diet.

diet may lower your risk of blood pressure, prevent type 2 diabetes, and reduce your risk of stroke and heart disease. The high fiber content of plant-based foods will allow you to eat more with fewer dense calories, which may help with maintaining a healthy weight. This antioxidant-rich diet may also decrease your risk of cancer and Alzheimer's disease. Many athletes have found that a plant-based diet increases endurance and allows for better physical performance. Eating this way will not only benefit your health, but it will also protect the environment by lowering your carbon footprint, saving the lives of animals, and keeping the air that you breathe while running cleaner.

Antioxidants

Free radicals are molecules produced by environmental toxins (e.g., ultraviolet light, pollution, and smoke) and your body's breakdown of what has been ingested. Free

Food Sources of Antioxidants

- Whole grains: brown rice, quinoa, farro, and oatmeal
- Beans: garbanzo, lentil, black, and edamame
- Nuts: raw, unprocessed, such as almonds and walnuts
- Seeds: hemp, pumpkin, flax, sesame, and chia
- Herbs/spices: turmeric, garlic, ginger, and cayenne
- Fruits and vegetables with bright colors: leafy greens, peppers, berries, plums, and oranges

radicals damage your body's cells, potentially leading to disease. Antioxidants act as scavengers for free radicals, intercepting them and protecting you from disease-producing damage.

These powerhouse nutrients can be found in fruits, vegetables, whole grains, nuts, seeds, herbs, spices, and happily dark chocolate. Brightly colored fruits and berries contain vitamins A, C, and E, all of which function as important antioxidants.

Plant-Based Protein

Protein is essential to your health, as it provides the building blocks for our body tissues and repairs damaged tissue, particularly after a workout. The amount of protein needed is based on your body weight and level of activity. To calculate your recommended daily protein intake, multiply your weight in pounds by 0.36, and this will give you the amount of protein in grams per day. For example, to determine the daily protein needs of a 160-pound woman, you would use the following equation: $160 \times 0.36 = 57.6$. Excellent sources of plant-based protein include chickpeas, lentils, black beans, walnuts, and tofu.

Essential Fatty Acids (EFAs)

Omega-3 and omega-6 are polyunsaturated fats that are the building blocks of healthy cells. They are integral in the formation of the skin's oil barrier and keep your skin plump and hydrated.

Omega-3 fatty acids not only benefit your skin but also are useful to lower your risk of heart disease and joint pain. They have also been shown to slow the development of Alzheimer's disease. Dietary sources include walnuts, flax, avocados, oily fish, and eggs.

Omega-6 fatty acids are essential fats that provide energy. The body cannot make them, so they must be obtained through diet. Omega-6 fatty acids are common in processed foods. Dietary sources include almonds, walnuts, and oils, such as soybean, vegetable oil, and corn oil. One should consume more omega-3 than omega-6.

Vitamins and Minerals

Vitamins and minerals are essential for healthy skin as well as your general well-being. Although they can be taken in supplement form, it is better to obtain them from foods. The following are recommended, with guidelines for daily doses and the best sources to look for:

Check the daily values of your multivitamin and any supplements you take and add them up. Just as you do not want to get too little of a vitamin, it cam be dangerous to get too much.

• **Vitamin A** is an important nutrient for skin and eye health. It has two forms: retinoids and carotenoids. Retinoids are animal derived (liver, kidney, eggs, dairy). Carotenoids are plant derived (dark yellow vegetables, carrots, fruit). Retinoids aid in collagen production, stimulate cell turnover, and reverse and treat chronic sun damage, they are often found in skin-care products targeted for antiaging, sun damage, and acne. Topical vitamin A may initially irritate your skin and increase your sun sensitivity. Discuss its use with your dermatologist. Ingesting too much vitamin A can cause side effects, including headaches, blurred vision, and liver damage. The recommended daily allowance for vitamin A is 900 micrograms for men and 700 micrograms for women. Sweet potatoes, pumpkin, dark leafy greens, oily fish such as salmon, and eggs are excellent sources of vitamin A. Accutane is a synthetic vitamin A derivative that when taken by mouth is used to treat severe cystic acne.

• **Vitamin B$_3$** (niacin) is an antioxidant, water-soluble vitamin and one of eight B vitamins that form the B complex. There are two forms of B$_3$: Nicotinic acid may prevent heart disease by lowering LDL (bad) cholesterol and triglycerides and by raising HDL (good) cholesterol levels. Niacinamide plays a role in DNA repair and reduces the rate of nonmelanoma skin cancer, but it has not been shown to lower cholesterol levels. When used topically, niacin has an anti-inflammatory effect and can calm irritated skin. Niacin supplements may cause facial flushing. The recommended daily allowance for vitamin B_3 is 16 mg for men and 14 mg for women. Dietary sources of B_3 include peanuts, lentils, wild-caught salmon, brown rice, and mushrooms.

• **Vitamin C** is a powerful antioxidant that neutralizes disease-causing free radicals and also plays a role in the production of collagen, a basic protein from which the skin, hair, nails, tendons, and ligaments are made. This is why you will often find vitamin C in many anti-aging skin-care products. I recommend 1,000 mg per day for both men and women. Food sources include kale, broccoli, and citrus fruits such as oranges. Oral vitamin C can enhance the effectiveness of sunscreen.

• **Vitamin D** is actually not a vitamin; it is a fat-soluble hormone that helps to regulate the skin's immune function, decreases inflammation, and aids in skin cell turnover. It is sourced from our skin and our gut. Our gut absorbs vitamin D_2 (ergocalciferol) and D_3 (cholecalciferol) from dietary sources, and our dermis makes vitamin D_3 with the aid of UVB. Vitamin D also helps our bodies to absorb calcium. Once vitamin D is ingested into the gut or synthesized in the skin, it must then be activated in the liver and then in the kidneys in order for its benefits to be realized. The activated form of vitamin D, calcitriol, circulates in the blood, where it plays a role in many organ systems, including the bones, heart, brain, and skin, and in immune health. Very little vitamin D is stored. The amount of sunlight needed for the skin to make vitamin D is equivalent to 15 to 20 minutes of sunlight per day. Additional sun exposure without proper sun protection will increase your risk of skin cancer. The recommended daily allowance for vitamin D is 600 IU for both men and women. Dietary sources include oily fish such as salmon, egg yolks, and mushrooms. You can also drink citrus juice and milk fortified with vitamin D.

• **Vitamin E** is an antioxidant that neutralizes ultraviolet damage. Topical vitamins C and E work synergistically well together in skin care products. Using or applying a product that contains both vitamin C and vitamin E will provide more benefit than using a product that contains either one alone. Vitamin E is produced in the dermis by sebum, which helps to moisturize and lubricate the skin. Those with dry skin may benefit from increasing their dietary vitamin E intake or taking a supplement. The recommended daily dose of vitamin E is 15 mg for both men and women. Dietary sources include nuts and seeds such as almonds and sunflower seeds, avocados, and spinach.

Recommended Daily Requirements

Vitamin A	900 mcg/day for men; 700 mcg/day for women
Vitamin B$_3$	16 mg/day for men; 14 mg/day for women
Vitamin C	1,000 mg/day for both men and women
Vitamin D	600 IU/day for both men and women
Vitamin E	15 mg/day
Zinc	11 mg for men; 8 mg for women

- **Zinc** is a mineral required for DNA synthesis, wound healing, and immune function. It provides anti-inflammatory and antibacterial benefits. When used topically, zinc oxide is a physical sun protectant that deflects harmful ultraviolet rays, just like Wonder Woman's shield would do. Topical zinc creams can also be used in wound care (think burns or diaper rash) and to repair the important barrier function of the skin.

Our bodies do not store zinc, so daily supplementation is important. Dietary sources of zinc include oysters, pumpkin seeds, chickpeas, and beans. The recommended daily dose of zinc is 11 mg for men and 8 mg for women.

Water

Most people walk around in a state of dehydration. Especially when you are exercising and sweating, hydration is crucial to performance.

Water is not the only source of hydration. You can

hydrate with any noncaloric beverage, such as seltzer water with lime. Foods with higher water content, such as cucumber, watermelon, and celery can be used for variety.

In general, you should aim to drink half of your body weight in ounces. For example, if you weigh 160 pounds, you should drink 80 ounces of hydrating fluid each day to maintain your level of hydration.

A quick way to monitor your level of hydration is to look at your urine. Urine should be light yellow. Dark urine is a sign of dehydration. Another sign of dehydration can be hunger, and people eat when what they really need to do is drink.

Drinking more water, especially during a race, can cause your electrolytes, particularly your sodium levels, to be diluted. This is called hyponatremia, and it can be very dangerous. Symptoms of this are excessive fatigue, dizziness, and confusion. If you sweat profusely, are running in a hot and humid environment, or running/training for more than an hour, replace electrolytes during hydration by drinking products like Powerade or Gatorade, rather than drinking plain water. It can also help to eat a salty snack, such as pretzels on a long run.

Chapter 3

CBD (Cannabidiol) and the Athlete

How Does CBD Help the Athlete?

Through exercise and training, all athletes, whether they are amateurs or professionals, place stress on the body, most notably on the muscles, joints, and skin. This wear and tear causes inflammation, which in turn leads to injury. Chronic use of nonprescription pain relievers, such as NSAIDs (naproxen sodium and ibuprofen), can cause kidney damage and potentially increase risk for stroke and cardiac events. Chronic use of prescription pain relievers can lead to addiction and overdose. While direct clinical studies of CBD use in athletes are unavailable at this time, information available on nonathletes can be extrapolated to the athlete population.

What Is CBD?

CBD is one of more than 100 naturally occurring compounds found in a group of flowering plants called *Can-*

The Confusion

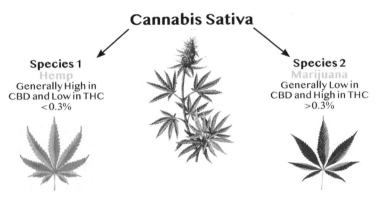

CANNABIS SATIVA HAS TWO SPECIES

Cannabis Sativa

Species 1
Hemp
Generally High in
CBD and Low in THC
<0.3%

Species 2
Marijuana
Generally Low in
CBD and High in THC
>0.3%

nabis sativa. THC (tetrahydrocannabinol) is the most notorious of the compounds because of its psychotropic effects, or "high," when used. On the other hand, CBD and the many non-THC compounds derived from the *Cannabis sativa* plant have the potential to offer many medicinal benefits without the high.

How Does CBD Work?

To understand how CBD works in our bodies, we must first understand how our cells function. Our cells communicate with each other through a complex cell messenger or signaling system. Cells can change their behavior based on the message they receive. The message (key) is received by a receptor (lock) located on the cell. When the key fits in the lock, the behavior of the cell can change. This complex signaling system, which was discovered in the 1990s, is called the *endocannabinoid system* (ECS). It plays a role in regulating many of our bodily functions related to our overall health and sense of well-being, including sleep, mood, and pain, Additionally, it regulates immune, skin, and nerve function.

The ECS has three components:

- *Endocannabinoids* are neurotransmitters (messengers) that are produced by our bodies and interact with receptors to keep our body functioning properly. Omega-3 and omega-6 fatty acids are important in our body's production of endocannabinoids. *Phytocannabinoids* are plant-derived sources, including CBD and THC, that function similarly to our bodies' endocannabinoids.
- *Receptors* bind endocannabinoids. They are scattered throughout our bodies and function as a lock. Cannabinoids act as the key.
- *Enzymes* help to make and then break down the endocannabinoids.

The ECS described previously opens the door to the following potential benefits of CBD for the athlete:

- Calms anxiety, which plays a role in race performance
- Provides nonsteroid anti-inflammatory relief to manage training injuries
- Improves sleep
- Calms gut discomfort

How CBD Benefits the Skin

- Provides anti-inflammatory/antioxidant properties
- Neutralizes damage from environmental free radicals
- Minimizes oil production

Is CBD Legal?

Since 2018, the World Anti-Doping Agency no longer prohibits the use of CBD, and the World Health Organization categorizes CBD as safe and well tolerated in humans. However, THC is still prohibited by these organizations.

The 2018 Farm Bill removed hemp as a controlled substance and legalized hemp cultivation with restrictions. CBD is legal federally, but federal guidelines dictate that it must be sourced from the hemp plant and contain less than 0.3 percent THC by dry weight. State laws may vary. For updated information on the laws of each state regarding CBD, go to https://www.safeaccessnow.org/states.

Hemp Oil versus CBD Oil

Both hemp and marijuana plant species have seeds, leaves, stalks, and flowers. Hemp seed oil is made only from hemp seeds. It is used in cooking and as a staple in skin-care products because of its non-pore-clogging properties.

CBD oil is made from the leaves, stalks, and flowers of the hemp plant, which contains a higher concentration of CBD than the marijuana plant, but is nonpsychoactive because it contains less than 0.3 percent THC.

CBD oil absorbs into the skin and binds to cannabinoid receptors in the body.

How to Use CBD and Dosing

Dosing approved by the Food and Drug Administration (FDA) is available only for Epidiolex, the one prescription

Other Terms You Should Know

- *Isolate*: Contains only CBD from the cannabis plant
- *Broad spectrum*: Contains other compounds and cannabinoids found in the plant, such as terpenes
- *Full spectrum*: Broad spectrum + low quantities of THC (less than 0.3 percent)
- *Terpenes*: Fragrant oils found in plants
- *Flavonoids*: Phytonutrients found in fruits and vegetables
- *Entourage effect*: Enhanced benefit of all components working together, as seen in a full-spectrum product

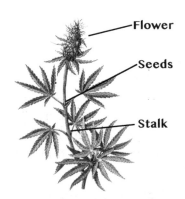

The Hemp Plant

Flower

Seeds

Stalk

CBD Oil

- Extracted from the whole hemp plan
- Low in THC
- Rich in CBD (cannabidiol)
- Contains additional cannabinoids, such as CBN, CBG, and CBC
- Primarily used for medical purposes

VS. Hemp Oil

- Extracted only from hemp seeds.
- No THC
- No CBD
- Rich on omega-3 and omega-6
- Primarily used in cooking, as a moisturizer, and as a daily supplement.

What to Look for in a CBD Product

- Derived from whole hemp, which is sometimes called "full spectrum"
- Certificate of analysis by an independent third party
- Consider products by Joyla™, which is a company that focuses on skincare for athletes, many of which contain CBD. Visit www.JoylaSkin.com for more detail about CBD and skincare products for athletes.

cannabis-derived product used for the treatment of seizures and epilepsy. No other products have official guidelines for usage. Before you start using any CBD product, it is recommended that you consult your doctor.

The dosage of CBD depends on the type of product and the way in which it is taken. CBD comes in many forms:

- Ingested: Capsules, gummies, pills, tinctures
- Topical: Muscle rubs, balms, creams, oils, lotion
- Inhaled: Vaping offers fast absorption, but inhaling any product comes with the risk of lung damage.

Look for products that have been tested by a third party to ensure the label's accuracy and certificate of analysis.

CBD should not show up on any drug test as long as you are purchasing third-party-tested CBD with no added THC. Because drug testing in professional athletes is often more sensitive, they could potentially test positive for trace amounts of THC if using CBD products.

Chapter 4
Sun Protection

As a 10-time marathoner, I much prefer running outdoors than inside on a treadmill. I enjoy the scenery, camaraderie, and fresh air—with the exception of humidity. However, I also recognize the increased risks associated with prolonged outdoor activities. I advise my patients that they have earned the right to enjoy their outdoor activities, but I want them to do it safely.

Sunscreen

Using sunscreen is an important component of your sun-protective routine. Regular and proper sunscreen use can decrease your overall risk of skin cancer and protect skin from premature aging, wrinkle formation, and discoloration. Sun damage accumulates over your lifetime, so everyone over the age of six months, regardless of skin color, should incorporate the use of daily sun protection.

The sun creates UV radiation as natural energy that is divided into three categories (UVA, UVB, and UVC). All light is found on the electromagnetic spectrum and is measured in nanometers (nm). Because UV light has shorter wavelengths, you cannot see it, but your skin can feel it and be damaged by it. Each form of ultraviolet light can damage your skin's DNA and is associated with the development of skin cancer.

UVA (315–400 nm) penetrates deeply and is associated with skin aging and wrinkling. It can penetrate windows and clouds. This is the main wavelength used in tanning beds. *Broad-spectrum* is the term used on sunscreen indicating protection against UVA rays. There is no rating system for UVB or UVC.

UVB (280–315 nm) is responsible for suntan and sunburn. UVB rays can be filtered and do not penetrate glass. *SPF* is the term used on sunscreen indicating protection against UVB rays.

UVC (100–280 nm) is the most damaging, but fortunately, these rays do not penetrate the ozone layer and pose less of a risk for skin cancer development. They can be produced by some manmade sources, such as UV sanitizing bulbs. There is no rating system for UVC protection.

Sunscreens contain ingredients intended to prevent the sun's UV rays from contact with your skin. There are two categories of sunscreens:

• **Physical sunscreens** act like a deflecting shield to scatter and block the sun's rays before they can penetrate into your skin. They contain minerals such as zinc oxide and titanium dioxide.

- **Chemical sunscreens** work like sponges to absorb UV rays before they penetrate into your skin. They contain ingredients such as avobenzone, oxybenzone, octisalate, homosalate, and octinoxate.

UV Rays and How They Affect Skin

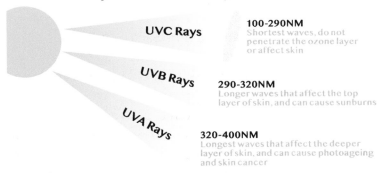

UVC Rays

100-290NM
Shortest waves, do not penetrate the ozone layer or affect skin

UVB Rays

290-320NM
Longer waves that affect the top layer of skin, and can cause sunburns

UVA Rays

320-400NM
Longest waves that affect the deeper layer of skin, and can cause photoageing and skin cancer

Wavelengths of ultraviolet (UV) rays are measured in nanometers (NM), or billionths of a meter.

How to Choose a Sunscreen

Sunscreen versus Sun Block

The terms *sunscreen* and *sun block* have been used interchangeably, but the difference lies in the way they protect your skin. Sun*screen* is similar to the screen in a window in that it allows some sun to penetrate. These products are also known as chemical sunscreens and contain compounds that absorb UVB light. A sun ***block*** functions as a physical block, like a wall that blocks penetration of UV light. The term *sun block* can be confusing as it provides a false sense of security that it offers complete protection. Physical blockers are often better tolerated on sensitive skin. They also tend to leave a white cast on darker skin.

SPF

SPF stands for **S**un **P**rotection **F**actor. It measures the length of time it would take for UVB rays to burn your skin. For example, if your skin would normally turn red when exposed to the sun in one minute, after you apply an SPF 30 product, your skin would turn red in 30 minutes. You will still get the same amount of damage, but it will just take you 30 times as long to do so. SPF only refers to UVB. There is no rating system for UVA or UVC. For protection against UVA rays, you should look for products that specifically state UVA/UVB protection or broad spectrum. As a dermatologist, I recommend for daily use—days when you are going to school or work, running errands, and so forth—an SPF of 30 or greater. If you will be spending a longer period of time outdoors—days when you are running, playing tennis, or sitting through a baseball game—start with a minimum SPF of 50 or greater.

Manufacturers determine the SPF based on experiments conducted under controlled conditions in a lab. That means for you to get that same SPF, you have to apply the same amount of protection used in the lab testing. Most people don't use nearly enough. Ideally sun protection should be applied to every inch of sun-exposed skin 20 minutes before your outdoor activity. To cover the face, arms, ears, neck, chest, and legs, the average adult should use a full ounce of sun protection. That is roughly a shot glass full. Let's do the math. Most drugstore containers of sun protection contain 8 to 12 ounces. If you're applying enough protection each day of outdoor training and reapplying every 2 to 3 hours, then these bottles should last you no more than a week. On a weekend at the beach, you should go through an entire bottle of sunscreen. If not, you are not getting the SPF you think you are. If you should be applying a shot glass full of sun protection, but you apply a nickel full, you are probably only wearing SPF 5. Apply a full ounce (shot glass full) every two to three hours to ensure you are receiving proper protection. Most people fail to apply enough and/or fail to reapply often.

Don't forget your lips! Statistically, women have a lower incidence of skin cancer of the lip, likely because of lipstick wearing. Opaque lipsticks often contain zinc

Dr. Brooke Derm Tip

Sun Protection Product Recommendations for Lips

- ChapStick Sun Defense SPF 25
- Aquaphor Lip Protectant + Sunscreen Lip Balm
- Joyla™

oxide, which is a physical sun blocker. Lipstick is attractive and functional. Avoid lip gloss, which is like baby oil for your lips, making you more likely to burn.

Lotion, Spray, Gel, Wipe, or Stick?

This is a question of preference of texture and convenience. Whether you use creams, lotions, or sprays doesn't matter—as long as you are using a sufficient amount.

If you choose a spray, understand that spray-on products are aerosolized droplets. Make sure to avoid inhaling and connect the dots by rubbing the product into your skin after spraying it in, which will avoid skipped areas. If you have oily, acne-prone skin, choose a sun protection with a lighter weight, such as a gel or spray. They are usually labeled as sports formulations. They may have a higher alcohol content and are less likely to occlude your skin. For dry, sensitive skin, consider a lotion formulation.

Sticks are convenient and perfect to carry with you

Dr. Brooke Derm Tip

What to Look for on a Sunscreen Label

- Broad spectrum
- SPF 30 or greater
- Sweat resistant

Note: Apply a full ounce 20 minutes before outdoor activity, and reapply every two to three hours while in the sun.

during training for easy, quick reapplication. They can also be used on the lips.

Sweat-proof or Waterproof?

To dispel a popular misconception, sun-protection methods are *not* sweat- or waterproof, despite product marketing information to the contrary. When you are swimming and notice the water around you becoming oil-slicked, you are actually seeing your sun protection wash away. No sun-protection product can be completely sweat-proof or waterproof. The appropriate labeling should state "sweat resistant" and "water resistant," and the label should state the length of time that you are protected. For example, a label that states "sweat resistant for 80 minutes" means that it will protect your skin for 80 minutes during a sweat-inducing activity. Keep an eye on the time and know that, depending on how fast you run or walk, you will need to reapply at that 80-minute mark to maintain your protection.

How Often Should I Reapply It?

Sunscreen wears off, washes off, and sweats off. That is why it is important to reapply your sun protection often. A good rule of thumb is to reapply sun protection every two to three hours.

Sun Protection Summary

The following guidelines will provide you with the best-possible protection for your skin:

- Avoid exercising outside during peak sun time, between 10 a.m. and 4 p.m.

- Wear sun protection every day. Put it on first thing in the morning. Use sunscreen with an SPF of at least 30.

- Apply sun protection at least 20 minutes before sun exposure, and reapply it every two to three hours.

- Apply enough sun protection to obtain the SPF rating for the product; the amount that is needed is stated on the label or packaging. Generally, 1 ounce, or shot glass full, is the amount of sunscreen that should be applied to exposed face, arms, and legs when you're wearing a tank and shorts for a run.

- Apply sunscreen during winter months as well.

- Sunscreen applied to your forehead can run into your eyes and sting. Wear a hat with a brim and sunglasses, and then apply sunscreen from below your eyes.

- Wear wicking clothing to cover up as much skin as possible (see "Clothing" on page 37).
- Wear sunglasses and a hat to protect your face (see "Sunglasses" and "Hat or Visor" below and on page 36).

Suggested Broad-Spectrum Sunscreen

- Joyla™ Be Protected Mineral SPF 30
- Blue Lizard SPF 30 Sport mineral-based sunscreen
- KINeSYS SPF 50 Fragrance Free Spray
- Neutrogena Ultra Sheer dry-touch SPF 100+
- Coppertone Sport SPF 50
- Colorescience Sunforgettable Total Protection Brush-On Shield SPF 50

Sun-Protective Clothing

Sun protection is far more than just sunscreen. When you are outdoors, not only can the sun's UV rays cause damage by direct absorption into the skin, but the skin is also damaged by UV rays reflected from surfaces such as concrete, water, and sand. So head-to-toe sun-protective measures are always important.

Hat or Visor?

Our head is the closest target of the sun's damaging rays. Wearing a hat is the first line of defense in protecting our scalp, hair, forehead, and eyes. Choose a hat made of tightly woven moisture-wicking technical fabric that can be easily

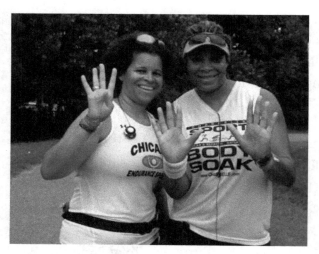

Sun protective running gear: With my running
buddy for life after a 14-mile training run.

washed. A hat is preferred over a visor as the hat will provide coverage for the scalp, which is particularly important
if your hair is thinning or you wish to protect the color of
your hair from fading. An adjustable Velcro closure will
allow flexibility with different hairstyles and head sizes. A
brightly colored hat with reflective trim will help to keep
you visible when running in low light conditions.

Coolibar Sunbreaker Running Cap has a removable
neck drape for added protection.

Sunglasses

Our eyes, especially our eyelids, are susceptible to damage from ultraviolet sunlight, which can increase the risk

of skin cancer. Prolonged sun exposure can also irritate the "whites" of our eyes, or conjunctiva; can damage the lens of the eye, leading to cataract formation; and can harm the retina, leading to a form of vision loss called macular degeneration. Prolonged exposure to elements such as wind and dry air can cause damage as well.

Choose polarized sunglasses that block UVA and UVB rays. The glasses should be comfortable, not too tight; cover your eyebrows; and have wide, wraparound arms to protect the skin of your temples.

Clothing

Wear moisture-wicking technical fabrics for your base layer. Clothing may have a UPF (ultraviolet protection factor) rating, which is similar to an SPF rating for sunscreens. UPF rating indicates what fraction of UV rays penetrate a particular fabric. A UPF 50, for example, means that the material allows one-fiftieth, or 2 percent, UV penetration, so it is theoretically 98 percent protective. Clothing with a UPF rating of 15 or greater earns the Skin Cancer Foundation's Seal of Recommendation. Clothes with UPF ratings below 15 are not considered sun protective. A 100 percent cotton T-shirt offers

Dr. Brooke Derm Tip

Add SunGuard to your laundry; it will provide a UPF 30 for up to 20 washings. Visit SunguardUV.com.

a UPF of 5. What we don't know is how long the UPF rating is maintained after washing and wear and tear.

Wisely chosen clothing offers long-lasting physical protection from ultraviolet damage. When more of your

Dr. Brooke Derm Tip

Head-to-Toe Sun-Protection Checklist

- Broad-spectrum sunscreen SPF 50+ applied 20 minutes prior to run
- UPF-protective clothing
- Polypodium leucotomos is a supplement made from ferns, which offers sun protection. I recommend it for all of my sun-exposed people.
- If you have sensitive skin, choose a mineral sun protection rather than a chemical one.
- Use enough—a full ounce (shot glass full)—to cover all sun-exposed body parts.
- If you are using your sun protection properly, an 8-ounce tube should be GONE after a weekend at the beach!
- Reapply every two to three hours.
- Don't forget your lips, ears, and back of neck, which are often-overlooked and easily burned areas.
- Wear a hat with a visor if you have thinning hair. Scalps burn too!

skin is covered, you are better protected. When UV rays hit your clothing, some of the rays penetrate through the clothing to your skin, some are reflected off, and some are absorbed by the fabric.

By adding a product called SunGuard to your laundry you can provide a UPF of 30 for up to 20 washings. Wash your hat, bra, runner's T-shirt, shorts, leggings, and socks with it. (For more information, go to https://store.sunguarduv.com.)

Polypodium Leucotomas Extract (PLE)

This dietary supplement from the tropical fern plant grown in Central and South America has been used for centuries because of its anti-inflammatory properties. Clinical research has demonstrated that, when taken orally, PLE provides some antioxidant and photoprotective properties. It is not an oral sunscreen. Topical sunscreen is the most effective method of sun protection we have. But no one is perfect in their application and reapplication of sunscreen. PLE can provide that extra layer of protection. It should be used in addition to properly applied topical sunscreen and photoprotective clothing. I recommend it for my patients who work outdoors, those who have a history of skin cancer or other conditions made worse by sunlight such as lupus or melasma or those who are taking medications that will make them more sensitive to sunlight. As with any supplement, please check with your doctor to determine if it is right for you.

Chapter 5
Skin Cancer

Running is a great way to improve overall health. However, if you enjoy exercising outside, as I do, then time in the sun, putting in all those miles training for a race, adds up and can potentially increase your risk for developing skin cancer. The effect of sun exposure over one's lifetime is cumulative, and it is this cumulative sun damage that will put you at risk for developing skin cancer.

Skin cancer is the type of cancer you can see. They generally do not hurt. It is the most commonly diagnosed cancer in the United States, with more than one million new cases diagnosed annually—more than all other types of cancer combined! According to the Skin Cancer Foundation, one in five Americans will develop skin cancer by age 70. Two people die from skin cancer every hour in the US.

Risk factors for developing skin cancer include:

- Fair skin
- Light-colored eyes and/or hair
- Family history of skin cancer

- History of blistering sunburns
- Tanning or tanning bed use
- Significant sun exposure as a child and young adult
- Numerous moles
- Chronic, non-healing wounds
- Prior radiation treatment to the skin
- Status of your immune system
- Your personal medical history

While you cannot control all of these risk factors, you can decrease your personal risk by incorporating sun-safe behaviors into your daily routine. When diagnosed and treated early, most skin cancers have an excellent survival rate.

Types of Skin Cancer

The three most common forms of skin cancer are basal cell carcinoma (BCC), squamous cell carcinoma (SCC), and malignant melanoma (MM). Skin cancers are classified as nonmelanoma skin cancers (NMSC = BCC, SCC) and Malignant Melanoma. They are named for the type of skin cells involved. If there is a suspicious lesion, a biopsy will be taken to confirm the diagnosis. A *skin biopsy* is an in-office procedure performed by your dermatologist using local anesthesia. The doctor will remove a small piece of the suspicious area and send it to a lab for testing. Treatment for NMSC usually involves an in-office surgical procedure to remove the growth and a small margin of the surrounding skin. Routine follow-up each year with a board-certified dermatologist is encour-

A board-certified dermatologist is a medical doctor who has completed specialized training in diseases of the hair, skin, and nails.

- 4 years college
- 4 years medical school
- 1 year internship
- 3 years residency
- + additional training

Look for the designation FAAD or AAD to assure you are seeing a board-certified dermatologist.

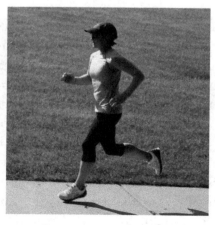

A sun protected runner

aged because, once you have had one skin cancer, the likelihood of developing others is very high. A trained dermatologist is likely to catch subtle, early changes. Most skin cancer deaths are from melanoma. Two of the most famous people who have had melanoma are Jimmy Carter and John McCain. It is a myth that people with dark skin do not get skin cancer. It's also untrue that only the elderly get skin cancer. My youngest skin cancer patient was a 24-year-old runner.

Basal cell carcinoma is the most common form of skin cancer and accounts for approximately 75 percent of all skin cancers. BCC develops from an abnormal growth of cells in the basal layer of the epidermis, typically after years of frequent sun exposure or tanning. Interestingly, BCCs are seen most frequently in outdoor athletes or people who work outdoors. Common locations for this type of skin cancer are the scalp, nose, ears, neck, and legs. They classically appear as small, pearly bumps with tiny blood vessels running through them. They may bleed on their own. When diagnosed and treated early, BCC is highly curable.

Squamous cell carcinoma develops in the squamous, or middle, layers of the epidermis. It is the second most common form of skin cancer, accounting for approximately 15 to 20 percent of all skin cancers. This type of skin cancer causes 15,000 deaths each year. SCC is characterized by well-defined, rough, thick, scaly lesions and plaques that may be painful and bleed. The most common areas are sun-exposed scalp, face, arms, and back. Smokers may develop SCC around their lips. With early diagnosis and treatment, SCC is highly curable. However, delay in treatment may result in the skin cancer spreading (metastasizing) to other areas of the body.

Malignant melanoma develops from abnormal growth of melanocytes (the cells that produce pigment) located in the lower portion of the epidermis. Although melanomas are less common and comprise only 5 percent of skin cancers, they are the leading cause of death from skin disease, with over 7,000 deaths annually in the US. Approximately 20 percent of melanomas develop from an existing mole. The remainder develop as a new spot on your skin. While the majority of melanomas develop in sun-exposed areas, they may also occur in other areas.

Melanomas are irregularly shaped and irregularly colored areas that may vary in size. Often, several different colors are seen within the lesion. Any lesion that changes rapidly should be examined carefully by a board-certified dermatologist. When you are looking at your moles, here are some general characteristics that should make you suspicious:

- Asymmetry—Two halves do not match.
- Borders are irregular.
- Color is changing, or there is more than one color within the mole.
- Diameter is larger than that of a pencil eraser.

- Evolving—The appearance is changing in size, color, shape, or behavior.

Skin Cancer in Skin of Color

While skin cancer occurs less frequently in people of color, when it does occur, it can be more deadly. This may be due to a combination of factors. It is not uncommon to delay seeking appropriate medical care because of the belief that people with darker skin do not get skin cancer. As a result, many patients with darker skin may not protect themselves from damaging UV rays. Genetics are also important to consider. Most people are actually a combination of two to four races. I have known some patients who, even though they may have a dark complexion, have northern European heritage and all of its associated risks, including a genetic predisposition to skin cancer regardless of their darker skin. In addition to genetics, immune status dictates the way in which your skin reacts to the sun. I have seen more skin cancers, even in my patients of color, in people who are taking medications to manage other medical conditions, such as HIV or lupus, or following an organ transplant. Such drugs may leave them immunosuppressed. If you have dark skin but also high blood pressure or diabetes, and you like to garden or run, not wearing sunscreen puts you at increased risk of skin cancer and skin discoloration.

More troubling is the fact that people of color tend to

develop squamous skin cancer (SCC) where the sun doesn't shine, such as the groin, buttock, and feet, as well as in areas of chronic skin trauma. Patients of color who have had lupus, for example, which often results in skin lesions, face an increased risk of developing skin cancer. The same holds true for those with burn injuries and non-healing wounds. When melanoma does occur in darker skin, it is most likely to occur on the hands and feet (acral lentiginous melanoma). Reggae legend Bob Marley died of a melanoma on his foot.

I had an African American woman come to me as a new patient. She had a spot on her temple that was not healing after a reasonable amount of time (2-4 weeks) and with no history of trauma. She had been advised by others to use a variety of treatments for eczema and ringworm that had not resolved the issue. I performed a biopsy of the area and diagnosed basal cell carcinoma.

The point is to know your body. For example, if you have a bug bite, scratch, or pimple, you know that it should probably heal in a week or two as long as you do not pick at it. If a month or two months have passed, or the lesion has healed but is now starting to bleed for no reason, this is abnormal and you should consult your board-certified dermatologist for evaluation.

Skin Cancer Risk Factors

The following factors will put you at increased risk of skin cancers (not all inclusive).

- Exposure to UV light (from sunlight or tanning)
- Fair skin, light hair (blonde, red)
- Precancerous lesions (actinic keratosis for SCC)
- History of skin cancer
- History of thermal burns or radiation therapy
- Weakened immune system
- Organ transplantation
- Human papillomavirus, a.k.a. HPV (SCC)

Dr. Brooke Derm Tip

- Examine your birthday suit on your birthday to familiarize yourself with your skin.
- Know what your moles look like, and look for any changes in size, color, or behavior, and note if you have new lesions.
- A "pimple" or "bug bite" should heal within a week or so. If it is not healing, or it's bleeding or growing, see a doctor. Recognize when your body is not behaving as it should, just as you do when you think you have a sprain or a shin splint.
- Get an annual skin cancer screening by a board-certified dermatologist, who can look at the small nuances and pick up early warning signs. The earlier the diagnosis, the better the prognosis.

- Arsenic/well-water exposure
- Chronic, nonhealing wounds
- Smoking (SCC)

Malignant Melanoma risk factors:

- Exposure to UV light
- More than 50 moles
- History of atypical (dysplastic) mole
- First-degree relative with melanoma
- Fair skin, light hair, light eyes
- Personal history of melanoma
- Weakened immune system

Dangers of Tanning

There is nothing healthy about tanned skin. Tanned skin, whether achieved by sunbathing or from frequenting a tanning salon, is unhealthy. Both activities provide sources of UV radiation and increase your risk for developing skin cancer. The World Health Organization (WHO) has placed tanning devices in the same cancer-causing category as tobacco. Those who utilize tanning beds are 60 percent more likely to develop malignant melanoma in their lifetime. I have had patients who insist on getting a "base tan" before they go on vacation in an effort to prevent a sunburn. I tell them that this in analogous to taking the batteries out of your smoke detector and thinking your house will not catch on fire. *Tanned skin is damaged skin.* Your melanocytes (see Chapter 1) produce more pigment in response to UV damage as a way to protect you. At some point, your body will not be able to correct the chronic damage, and the UV insult to your cells will progress to skin cancer. If you insist on being tan, consider self-tanners. I have yet to meet a patient older than 40 who does not regret tanning in their teens and twenties, whether that is because they have aged prematurely or because they now have skin cancer.

Age is a factor with everything. The longer you are on this earth, the more likely it is that something will go wrong with your health. But I am seeing younger and younger patients with skin cancer. The number of years you have been sun exposed (or a runner, boater, or golfer) is correlated with an increased risk of cancer.

I recommend a yearly full-skin examination by a board-certified dermatologist, who will evaluate and possibly biopsy any suspicious lesion. (Check out the American Academy of Dermatology website for more information: www.aad.org.) When educating my patients, I suggest they take a good look at their skin monthly to note any growths that are present or changing in color, size, or behavior (such as not healing properly or bleeding). Remember, with early diagnosis and treatment, skin cancer is entirely treatable.

Chapter 6

Common Skin Conditions in Runners

Acne

Any sweat-inducing activity creates a perfect storm for acne to occur: heat + moisture + bacteria. Commonly affected areas include the face, chest, and back. Hormonal shifts may cause acne to flare. While it may be tempting to pick at acne, avoid doing so as it may cause discoloration.

To minimize your chances of getting acne:

• Remove your makeup before a run. Makeup forms an occlusive barrier over your skin.

• Lighten up your sunscreen texture. Choose a gel lotion, or spray over a cream if you are acne prone (sports formulations) (see "How to Choose a Sunscreen" on page 29).

• Avoid non-breathable fabrics.

- Hit the showers. Try to bathe and wash your face as soon as possible after a workout. If you cannot get to a shower, keep Joyla™ BeFresh Wipes handy.

If you do get acne, consult with your board-certified dermatologist, who will customize a treatment plan for you. It is important to share that you are an outdoor athlete as this may alter the treatment plan.

Athlete's Foot

This superficial fungal infection thrives in moist, dark environments (your sweaty feet covered by socks and shoes). Wearing wicking technical fabric socks to wick the sweat from your feet should take care of it. Remove those shoes and socks as soon as possible after a run. Over-the-counter Lamisil cream works in most cases, but you may need prescription treatment. If athlete's foot is persistent, see your dermatologist. Apply the cream to the entire area a sock would cover and between toes.

Bloody Nipples

This condition is primarily seen in men and is caused by friction from a T-shirt rubbing against the nipples, creating irritated raw skin which may bleed—not a pretty sight for those postmarathon photos! To prevent it, avoid cotton T-shirts, wear a tech fabric, and lubricate your nipples with Vaseline or Body Glide before you run. You can also purchase a product called NipGuards online.

Folliculitis (*Malassezia* or *Pityrosporum Folliculitis*)

Folliculitis is very common among athletes and is due to the overgrowth of yeast within the hair follicle. Yeast and bacteria are normal inhabitants of our skin, but heat, moisture, and occlusion promoted by a sweat-inducing workout create a prime environment for the yeast and bacteria to thrive.

To prevent it, make your environment less hospitable. Wear clothing made of moisture-wicking fabrics. Keep a clean shirt in your car and change into it after your workout. Shower off as quickly as possible after exercising. If you can't get to a shower, clean off with Joyla™ BeFresh Wipes.

Foot Blisters

Foot blisters may be caused by friction, usually from new shoes, sweaty feet, and cotton socks. Try lubricating your toes with Vaseline or Body Glide, then use socks made of moisture-wicking technical fabric, such as COOLMAX or Dri-FIT. You should get your race-day shoes two to four weeks *before* the big race, and make sure you do your last few long runs in them. If you do get a blister close to race day, drain it by running a pin or needle through alcohol or a flame and then poke the blister. Let the fluid drain. Avoid removing the skin, which functions as nature's bandaid. Dr. Scholl's Blister Cushions from the drugstore can be helpful.

Friction/Chafing

Friction or chafing occurs in areas where skin rubs or bunches on skin, such as the inner thighs and underarms, and can be exacerbated by moisture and sweat. It can also be caused by an object, such as your fanny pack, water belt, sports bra, or new clothing that rubs or bunches as you run. For prevention tips, see "Bloody Nipples" on page 51. And do not wear new clothes or use new gear on race day (more on this subject in Chapter 9). Avoid having your water bottle/fanny pack directly on skin. Always place it over a shirt.

Frostbite

I love winter running, particularly in fresh snow, however cold temperatures can be dangerous. This tissue injury is due to extreme cold and is commonly seen on the hands, feet, nose, ears, and cheeks. Low temperatures and wind chill are primary risk factors. Typically, one will experience a burning sensation followed by numbness of the involved area. Heeding weather warnings, wearing appropriate layers, and limiting time outdoors will minimize the risk of frostbite. If it should occur, seek warm shelter and rewarm yourself with a warm shower and heating pads until the color of your skin returns to normal and the numbness resolves. Seek medical attention if your skin color or sensation does not return. The National Weather Service has created a wind chill chart that estimates the amount of time you can be exposed at different temperatures prior to the onset of frostbite (see https://www.weather.gov/safety/cold-wind-chill-chart).

Purple Toes

Also known as a subungual hematoma, I have had my share. This is a bruise under your toenail caused by friction, pressure, and trauma to the nail. Prevent it by making sure your shoes fit properly. Generally, your running shoes will be ½ to 1 size larger than your street shoes. There should be one thumb's width space from toe tip to shoe tip. You may also look for a more square-shaped toe box in the shoe so that the shoe is actually deep enough to accommodate your toes to wiggle. Lubricate your toes prior to running with Vaseline, and wear socks made of moisture-wicking material. If you do get a hematoma, you will likely lose your toenail, which you will survive, and it makes a great marathon story. Your toenail will grow back, but it will likely take several months. The bruise under the nail should grow out with the nail. Please consult a dermatologist or podiatrist if the nails is not growing out or if the discoloration of the nail expands and/or involves the skin around the nail.

Sunburn

The bright red hue you get from staying out in the sun too long is a sign that the skin is damaged. Sunburn is your body's alarm system; your body is telling you it has had too much. Brown skin can burn too! When you put raw meat on the grill, what happens? You are either panfrying (burn) or slow roasting (suntan), and either way you are getting cooked. More worrisome is the risk of skin cancer. Studies have shown that marathoners and outdoor athletes have a higher risk of malignant melanoma.

If you have a sunburn:

- Remove yourself from direct sun exposure and stay in a cooler (air- conditioned) environment.
- Take a cool shower or an oatmeal bath and apply cool compresses or refrigerated aloe gel to the area.
- Put on loose clothing.
- Take an anti-inflammatory as directed (ibuprofen or aspirin) if appropriate to relieve your discomfort.
- Stay hydrated. Remember, your skin is a barrier that maintains your body's hydration level. When the skin is compromised, it will not function well (see Chapter 1: Skin Function).
- Seek medical attention if sunburn covers a large portion of your body and/or you develop a high fever, chills, and pain.

To prevent future sunburn:

- Avoid running between 10 a.m. and 4 p.m.
- Wear a hat and sunglasses.
- Keep your clothes on. Men should keep their shirts on while running, and women should avoid running just in bra tops. Wearing some sort of sun protection from your clothes is the best way to prevent sunburn. Look for running clothing that offers UV protection, or wear darker colors, which block more UV rays than light colors.
- Apply a full shot glass (1 ounce) of broad-spectrum sunscreen SPF 50+ and reapply it every two to three hours.
- Look for shaded-area running routes.

Windburn

Windburn is most commonly seen in winter warriors. When exposed to cold, windy climates, like Chicago, you will undoubtedly experience dry, chapped skin. Apply a thin layer of Vaseline to any exposed area (face, lips). Wearing sunglasses or goggles and a gaitor will go a long way to protecting your skin from the elements. As with any concern, seek medical attention when necessary.

Chapter 7
Hair Care for the Athlete

As a physician, I teach my patients about the many benefits of exercise for one's mental and physical well-being. As an African American everyday athlete, I also understand that in order to reap the benefits of regular exercise, I must find additional time in my already-busy schedule to care for my hair. This means avoiding some hairstyles, such as blowouts, which will not last more than a day, and choosing a hairstyle that will look professional but require minimal maintenance between washings. Unfortunately, making this choice has cost some women their jobs. A news anchor in Mississippi was fired when she wore her hair in a natural style on the air. A middle-school girl was sent home from school for wearing braids, prompting a civil rights lawsuit. The CROWN Act (Creating a Respectful and Open World for Natural Hair) is a law introduced in California in 2019 that prohibits race-based hair discrimination, which is the denial of employment and educational opportunities because of hair texture or protective hairstyles, including braids, locs, twists, or bantu knots. (See thecrownact.com for more information.)

Published clinical studies document that African American woman may avoid physical activity because of its undesirable effect on their hair. More than 50 percent of African American women over the age of 20 are obese, leading to a higher incidence of diabetes and heart disease in this demographic. For many, it becomes a choice between health and hair.

Hair care differs based on texture. Straight hair tends to be oilier and should therefore be washed every one to three days. The curlier your hair is, the drier it is and should be washed less frequently. People with wavy hair should wash every 3 to 5 days, and those with curly and tightly coiled hair should wash every seven to fourteen days. Curly and coiled hair needs moisture and is prone to breakage. Sweat can cause the scalp to be damp, which can be the death of a blown-out style. When left on the scalp, salt, which precipitates from sweat, can make the skin itchy as it dries and cause hair breakage.

The following tips can help you maintain healthy hair:

• Avoid styles that prevent access to your scalp, weaves. Alternate washing with gentle shampoo with co-washing (rinsing with conditioner).

• Wash your hair on a regular basis with a gentle shampoo followed by a conditioner made for your hair texture.

The outer limit for hair washing is 14 days. You cannot wash your hair less frequently and not have a problem.

- Avoid styles that cause tension at the hair follicle (braids or weaves that are too tight, ponytails). This can lead to a type of hair loss called *traction alopecia*, which may be permanent. You should never see little bumps

Protective Hairstyles

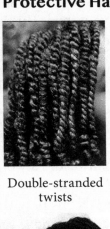

Double-stranded twists

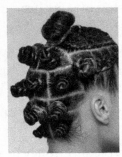

Bantu knots

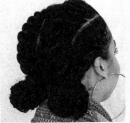

Crochet

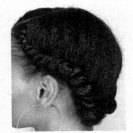

Cornrow

along the hair follicles after a style, and your hair should never be so tightly braided that it causes scalp pain.

- If you wear a headband, choose one with a satin or silk lining to prevent friction and breakage of hair along your hairline. Push the headband away from your forehead to avoid acne.

- UV light will fade hair color, so wear a hat.

- If you don't wear a hat, make sure to spray some sunscreen on the top of your head and in your part. This is a common site for sunburn. You can develop skin cancer on your scalp too!

- Avoid heat styling with blow-dryers and flat irons, which can damage already-dry hair.

- Moisturize your hair daily and see your stylist every 3 to 6 months for a trim.

- Apply a deep conditioner to your hair before a workout hair on wash day.

For any unresolved hair-related issues, consult with a board-certified dermatologist, who can diagnose and treat hair and scalp problems. (Visit the American Academy of Dermatology website for more information: www.aad.org.)

Chapter 8
Training Tips

As a 10-time marathoner who has coached thousands of novice runners and walkers to achieve their marathon goals, and as a dermatologist with many athletes in my practice, I want to share some training tips that I hope will get you to the finish line safely and without injury.

1. Get a checkup. Make an appointment with your primary care doctor to discuss your plans to run or walk. This is a good time to address and adjust for any health concerns that may affect your training, such as asthma, heart disease, pregnancy, diabetes, or arthritis.

2. Sign up for a race. Having a goal will help to keep you motivated.

3. Find a training partner or a group. These groups are invaluable for camaraderie, accountability, and safety. Your local running store can be an excellent resource for these groups. Others include jeffgalloway.com; blackgirlsrun.com; fleetfeet.com; and Road Runners Club of America (rrda.org).

4. Start where you are, and run your own pace. You will

find your pace. Running too fast for a distance will be unsustainable and cause frustration and injury.

5. Get properly-fitting shoes, and put a date on the box. Running shoes should last about 500 miles. Putting the date on the box will remind you when it is time to replace them. The support in the shoes will break down over time, making you susceptible to injury. You may need to insert orthotics in your shoes if you have flat feet. Running specialty stores such as Fleet Feet are a great resource to help you find the correct shot for your foot (size, support).

6. Choose your clothing wisely. A properly fitting running bra will support your breasts and minimize nipple irritation. Running stores such as Fleet Feet can help you select the best fit. Choose shorts that won't bunch when you run. I prefer bike shorts for this reason.

7. Cross-train and stretch. Any repetitive exercise can cause injury. Incorporating strength training, cross-training (adding another sport such as cycling), and stretching or yoga will maintain your flexibility and minimize overuse injuries. While training for my first marathon, I learned the hard way, after multiple injuries, that I should be stretching regularly. For subsequent marathons, I incorporated yoga two times per week and was able to get through a six-month marathon training period injury-free.

8. Stay hydrated. By the time you are thirsty, it is too late. Maintain a level of hydration daily. For proper hydration, the rule of thumb is to drink one-half of your body weight in ounces (if you weigh 150 pounds, for example, you should consume 75 ounces of hydrating fluid daily). Bring hydration with you on your runs in a fanny pack, or plan your course so that you have access to fluid. Chicago's lakefront is such a treat with water fountains interspersed along the way. Remember, too, that humid days can trick you. Minimize or avoid alcohol intake before long runs.

9. Run safely. Crimes against runners happen. Always be aware of your surroundings. Consider running with a group, especially if you run in isolated areas. When running alone, forgo the headphones. Run against traffic so you can see any cars coming toward you. Stay visible. When running at dusk, wear reflective running gear. Be tracked. Always let someone know where you are running and when you can be expected back. You can always use a running app and share your location with a friend. Carry some cash.

10. Wear sun-protective gear (see Chapter 4).

11. Have fun. Run happy. Run safe.

Chapter 9

Race Day Tips

You signed up for the race, pounded the pavement, logged those training miles, and now, with race day approaching, it is time to toe the line. Whether you are training for a 5K, marathon, or triathlon, here are a few tips to help you have a great race day.

1. Nothing new on race day. There is nothing worse than getting a rash or blister during your race from clothes or shoes. Training runs are meant to increase endurance for race preparation, but they should also serve as dress rehearsals for race day. Wear your race day gear to make sure those shorts and shirt don't bunch, wear that sports bra and make sure it fits well, and figure out the fit of the fanny pack to ensure it does not bother your lower back. If you are due for some new shoes, make sure you get them in time to take them on a few long runs prior to race day. For longer distances, try out your pre-race breakfast and race replenishments to make sure they are well tolerated and do not upset your stomach.

2. Apply and reapply sunscreen. Apply sunscreen on all exposed body parts 15 to 20 minutes before the race. If you are velocity challenged, as I am, and will be enjoying the marathon course longer than three hours, you will need to reapply your sun protection along the way. Put a small tube in your fanny pack or plan to have your support crew meet you along the course with your supplies. Make sure to cover your face, back of your neck, legs, arms, hands, chest, and lips (see "Head-to-Toe Sun-Protection Check-list" on page 38). Sunscreen is necessary even on a cloudy race day! If you are participating in a multisport race, reapply your sunscreen in the transition zone. Remember, sunscreen is not sweat-proof or waterproof.

3. Protect those peepers. Sunlight can damage the skin around your eyes and increase your risk of cataract formation. Look for wraparound sunglasses that block more than 99 percent of UVA and UVB rays. (This information will be on the sticker you peel off the sunglasses after you buy them.) Sunglasses should be worn even if you wear contact lenses.

4. Lube up what rubs. Friction is a runner's worst friend. And Vaseline petroleum jelly is a runner's best friend! Any body part that touches another body part should be lubed up as you get dressed for race day—this means inner thighs, upper arms, toes, bra straps, nipples, and waistbands. Now, about those nipples. This is a really common problem for men and women and the cause of the bloody T-shirt at the end of the race. Avoid those bloody shirts, guys! Use the lube. You might also try spot Band-Aids or NipGuards if needed.

5. Put your name on the front of your shirt. Who doesn't want the spectators shouting your name?

6. Be race-photo ready and have fun. Race photos are keepsakes and reminders of your accomplishments. Make sure to keep your race bib visible on the front of your shirt so the photographer knows who you are, and smile!

7. Know the race support. In the race instructions, it will tell you what support will be on the course so you can plan and prepare. Each race will tell you if they supply race support, what it is, and where it is located. For example: the race support includes Gatorade (vs Powerade) and water at every mile, GU and bananas at mile 18, and porta potties. This is important to know if you have not trained with what is offered, race day is not the time to try it. Either train with what is on the course, carry your own, or have your support crew meet you

8. Prepare your support team. Knowing your friends will meet you at mile 19 with smiles, a banana, and sunscreen can provide a much-needed boost.

9. Run happy. Run safe.

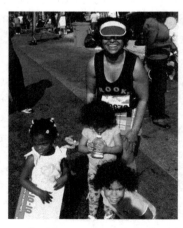

Support team: My kids meeting me at mile 25.

References

CBD-updated laws for each state:
https://www.safeaccessnow.org/states
Skin cancer information: aad.org; skincancer.org
2018 Farm Bill:
https://www.fda.gov/news-events/congressional-testimony/
hemp-production-and-2018-farm-bill-07252019
World Health Organization statement on CBD:
https://www.who.int/features/qa/cannabidiol/en/

Joyla™

BE WELL. BE FIT. BELONG.

Skincare Products and Training Resources
for the Everyday Runner

At Joyla™, we want all physically active people to enjoy their
lifestyle without the pain and discomfort often associated with
that active lifestyle. We believe that having the right products
and resources to aid in health and healing leads to better overall well-being and a simplified skincare regimen.

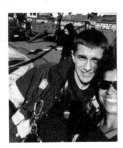

Photo of Dr. Jackson on the course at
the New York City Marathon with NYC's finest.

Acknowledgments

My village

I am forever grateful to my family, friends, and colleagues, who have encouraged and supported me on my running and publishing journeys!

My parents, Dr. Marvin and Aeolian Jackson, who taught me that with hard work and perseverance anything is possible.

Dave and Lisa Zimmer, who welcomed me into the Chicago running community and introduced me to my husband.

My husband, James, and our kids, Avery, Reese, and Myles, who make the marathon of life an adventure.

To Tracey, my partner in crime both on and off the trails.

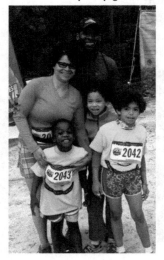

My family, running

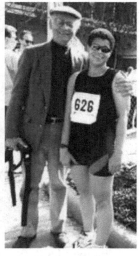

My dad met me at the finish line when I finished my first marathon.

About the Author

Brooke A. Jackson, MD, FAAD, is a board-certified dermatologist and dermatologic surgeon who takes a holistic approach when teaching and treating her patients about the importance of proper skincare. Her non-jargoned, relatable, and practical insights are welcomed by her patients. She specializes in creating customized and innovative treatment plans.

Dr. Jackson is a graduate of Wellesley College and Georgetown University Medical School. Upon completion of her internship at the University of Chicago and dermatology residency training at Henry Ford Hospital, Dr. Jackson became the first African-American dermatologist to be awarded laser fellowship training at Harvard University, where her interests and research helped to pioneer the uses of lasers in ethnic skin. Dr. Jackson completed a second fellowship in skin cancer surgery (Mohs) at Baylor College of Medicine In Houston, Texas, then joined the staff of the prestigious MD Anderson Cancer Center, where she founded the Mohs Surgery Unit and served as its director.

Having moved to Houston knowing no one, Dr. Jackson joined a running group to destress from the rigors of her medical training and ended up running her first marathon, and then another. She then relocated to Chicago, where she founded Chicago Fit, a marathon training group on the south side of Chicago focused on transitioning couch potatoes to marathoners. Under her leadership, that group grew from 40 members to over 400 in 4 years. Because of Dr. Jackson's community service to the running community, she was a featured runner on a billboard on I-94 for the 10-10-10 Chicago Marathon campaign. She met her husband at the Fleet Feet Running Store in Chicago, and they had their rehearsal dinner in the store on North Avenue.

In 2013, she and her family (husband, twin daughters, and a son) moved to the Raleigh/Durham area to be closer to Washington, DC, and care for her mother.

Dr. Jackson has published numerous articles, book chapters, and a CD-ROM relevant to her specialty. Because of her research interests and training, Dr. Jackson is a thought leader/expert in the field and lectures nationally and internationally on the use of lasers and cosmetic procedures in skin of color. She is also the author of *Child of Mine: Caring for the skin and hair of your adopted child.*

A gifted communicator, Dr Jackson has made frequent guest appearances on ABC, NBC, FOX, and WGN news regarding dermatologic issues, and she has been quoted in numerous national print publications, such as *Self, O, Runner's World, Essence, Ebony, Women's Day, Ladies Home Journal, Parenting, Teen Vogue,* and *Fitness* magazines.

An avid runner and budding triathlete, Dr Jackson has completed 10 marathons (26.2 miles) and 8 triathlons, and she was on the board of directors of Girls on the Run, an organization that encourages girls ages 8 to 12 to build self-esteem through running. She is also a frequent speaker for running groups on sun safety and skin cancer awareness.